BATHROOM STALL YOGA

by fitness trainer Grant Clark
and illustrator Rosie Kosinski

Foreword

Please enjoy the following series of movements to help restore balance to your body. Within the short amount of time required to complete these poses, you will stimulate blood flow, relax tensed muscles and focus on your body and breath, which aids in stress relief.

Rosie Kosinski was inspired by the yoga exercises that certified personal trainer and yoga instructor Grant Clark taught her. Grant curated the poses which are easily executed within any small spaces while offering the healing benefits of yoga.

• • •

Hands to Heart

This pose is a yoga staple and an excellent stance to begin any routine.

- Stand with your feet together or hip width apart.

- Bring your palms together in front of your chest.

- Focus on pushing your chest forward while simultaneously bringing the shoulders down and back.

- Press your feet into the ground, feeling the weight of your entire body.

- Stay here for 8 - 10 breaths, breathing deeply in and out of your nose.

Where: Shoulders, neck, chest and legs.

When: You are stressed and need a moment to recollect yourself and enjoy correct posture.

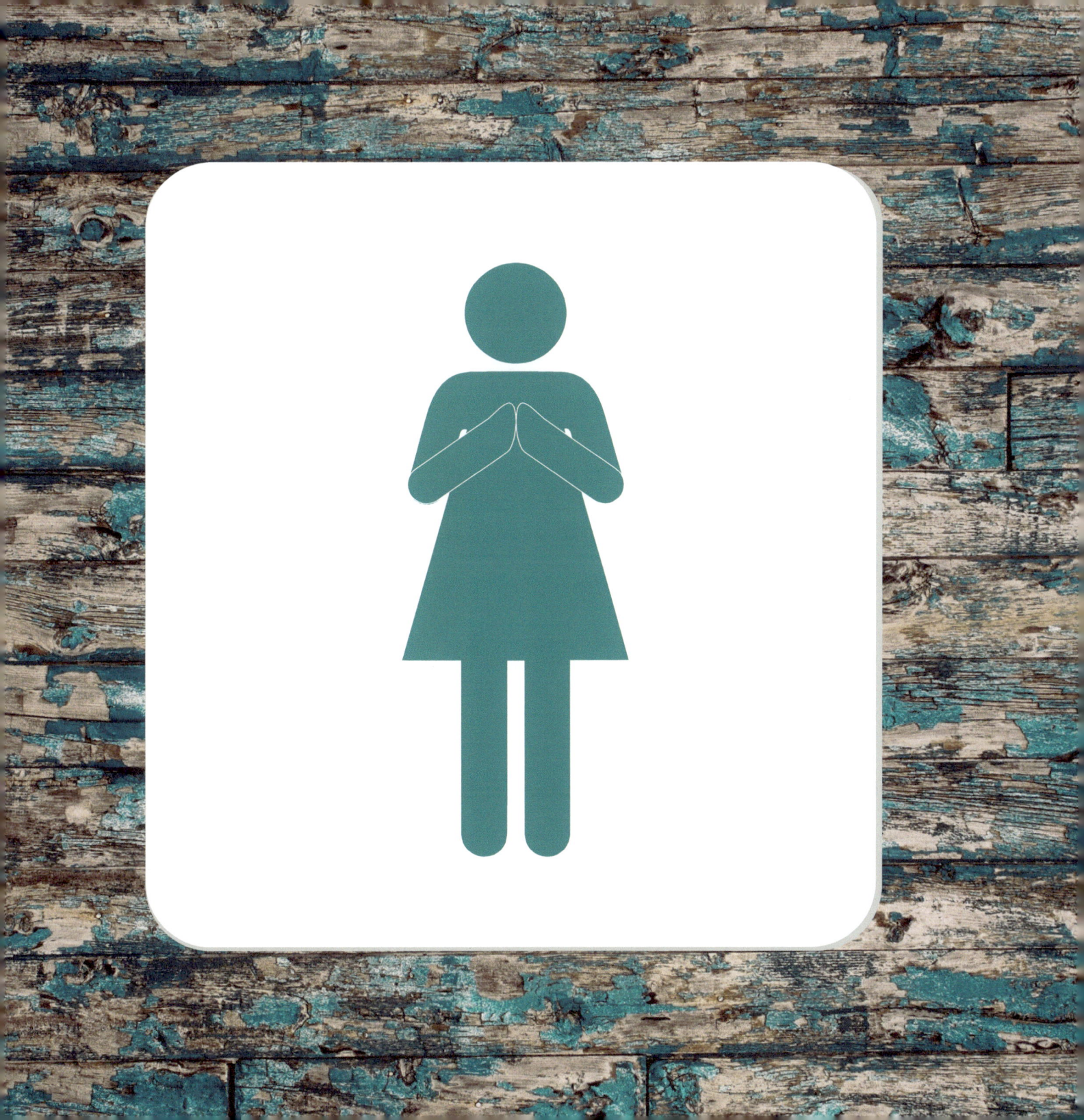

Shoulder Rotations

- Start with your chin down towards your chest and your shoulders rolled forward with your pinkies touching and your elbows connected.

- On an inhale, pull your arms back and push your chest forward, moving your head to look up towards the ceiling.

- Roll your shoulders down and back away from your ears.

- On your next inhale, return to the starting position.

- Complete 5 - 10 rounds, following your breath.

Where: Chest, upper back, neck and arms.

When: You feel tight from hunching over your desk.

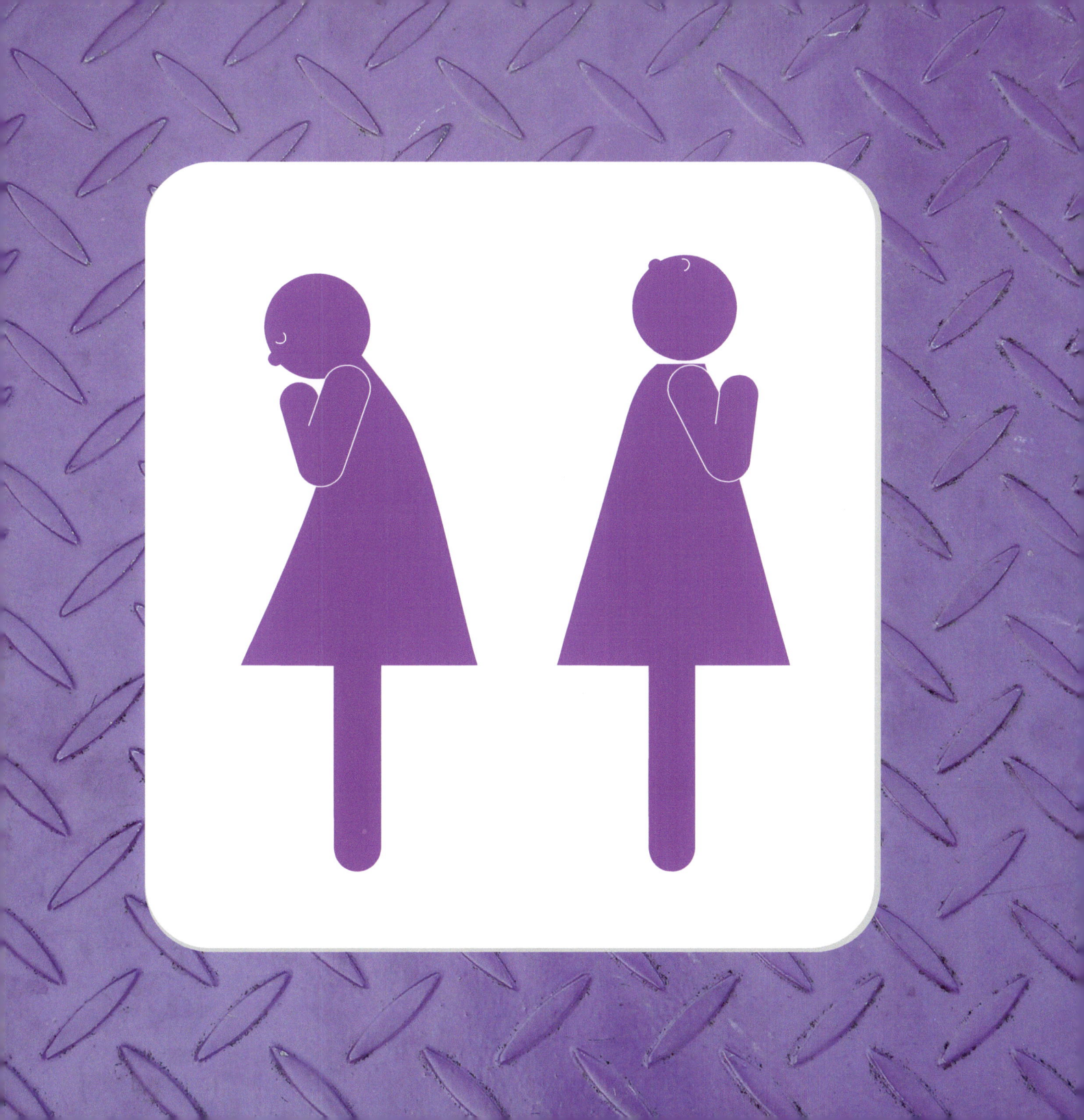

Neck Rolls

- Bring your palms together behind your back with your fingers pointing towards the floor.

- Roll your shoulders down and back away from your ears.

- Roll your head in large circles, focusing on bringing each ear to the nearest shoulder.

- Avoid constricting the bones in your neck by ensuring that your forehead does not face the ceiling.

- After 5 - 10 rotations, switch directions.

Where: Neck and shoulders.

When: Your neck is tight from looking down at a desk, device etc.

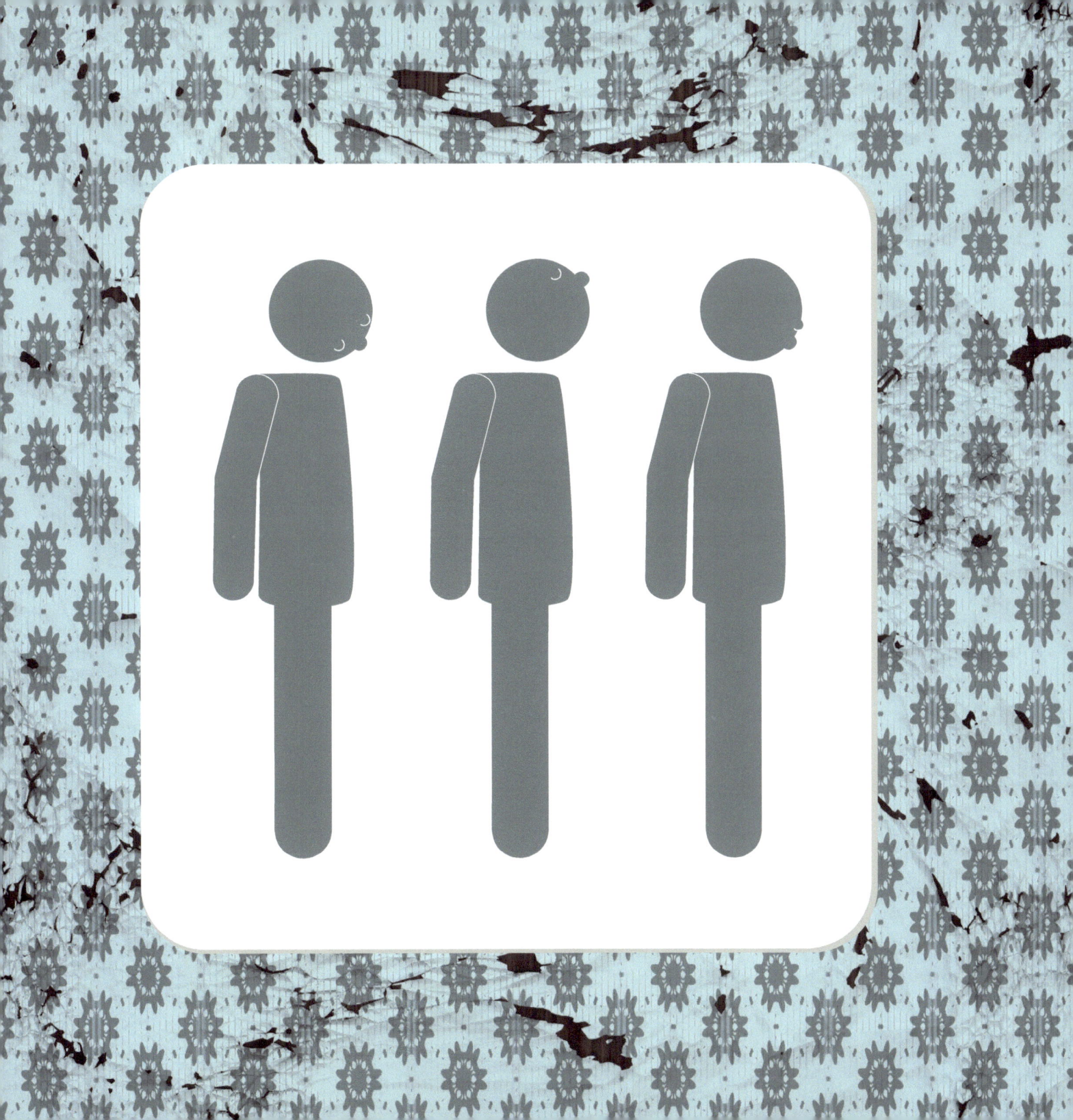

Standing Cat-Cow

- With your knees slightly bent, lay your palms on your thighs directly above the knees.

- On an inhale, bring your gaze to the ceiling, pushing your chest out and pressing your tailbone up to the sky to create an arch in your back.

- On an exhale, bring your chin to your chest and tuck your hips forward to form a C shape with your back.

- Repeat by following your breath for 5 - 10 rounds.

Where: Upper and lower back, hips, chest and neck.

When: You sat for 3 hours in a meeting.

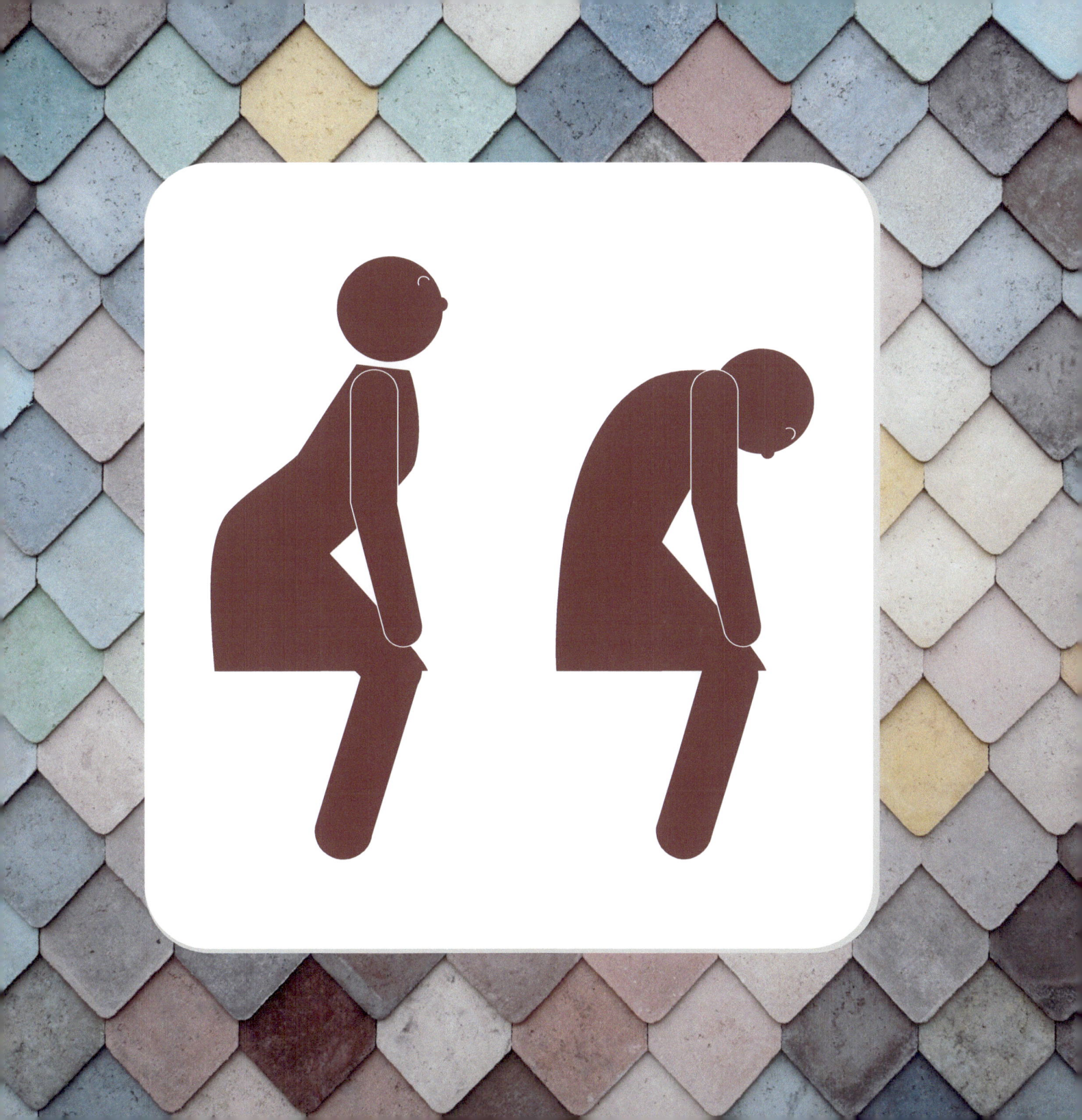

Crescent Moon

- With your feet together or hip distance apart, inhale your arms to the ceiling pressing your palms together.

- Press your arms upwards while pulling your shoulders down and back away from the ears.

- On your next exhale, lean your upper body to the right, allowing your head to relax in between your arms.

- Inhale back to center and on the next exhale, lean towards the left.

- Following your breath, move back and forth 5 - 8 times.

Where: The entire side of your body from your shoulders down to your hips.

When: You need to move in a new direction.

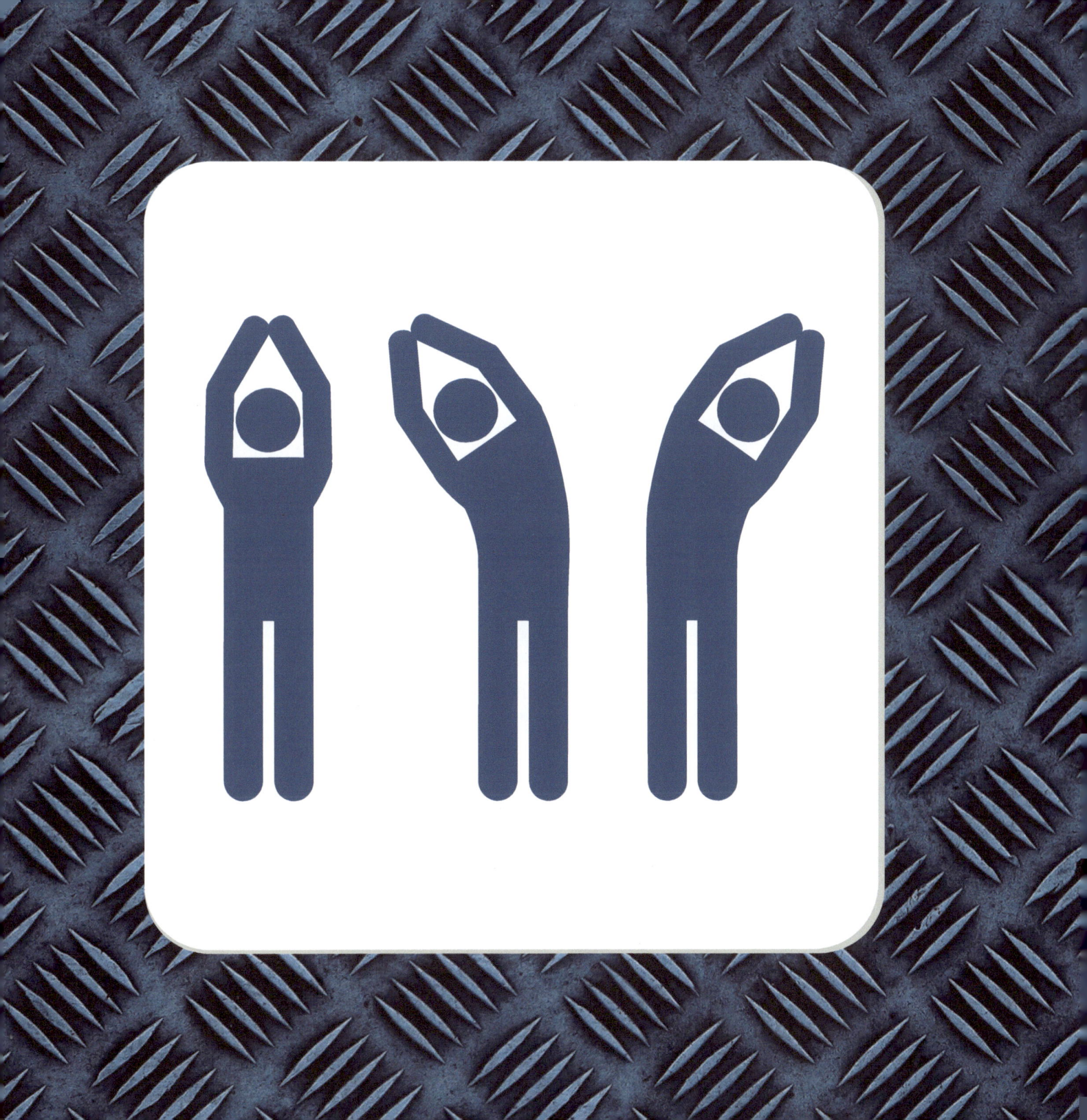

Victory Squat

- Place your feet a little wider than hip distance apart. Turn the feet out so they form a forty five degree angle.

- Align your shoulders and elbows on both sides with your arms up to form a U shape.

- On your next exhale, let out an audible 'ahh' and squat.

- Sit down into an imaginary chair while you lower your elbows down to your ribs.

- Complete 5 - 10 squats, each time letting out the audible 'ahh' sound.

Where: Hips, buttocks, legs.

When: You need energy and it is not quite time for your 2 o'clock coffee.

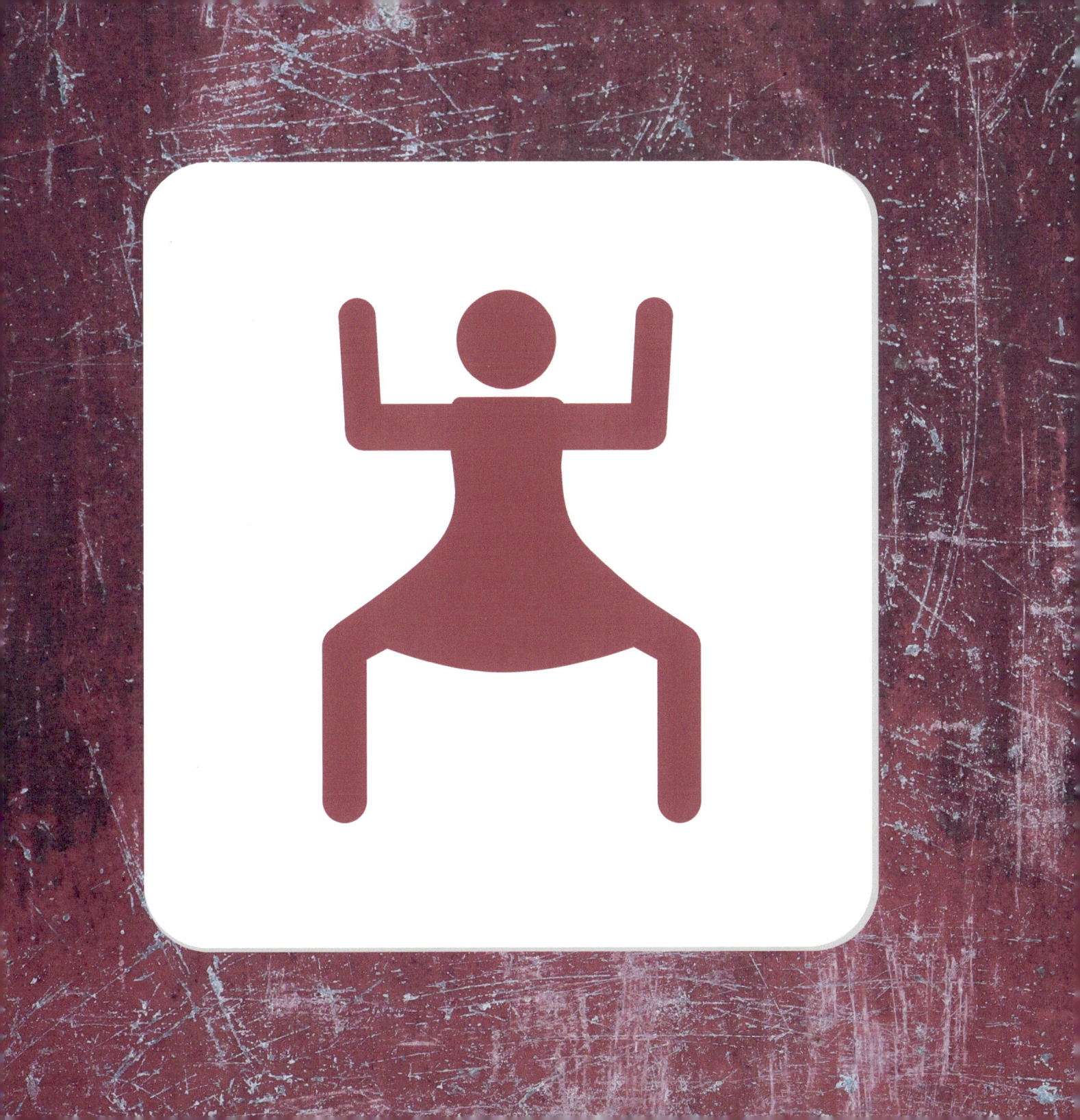

Standing Downward Dog

- Hinging at the hips, bring your chest parallel to the ground.

- Placing your hands, arms straight, on the wall in front of you.

- Bend your knees as much as necessary.

- Press your tailbone up in the air to create a straight back.

- Hold the pose for 5 - 10 breaths. Roll out of the pose by bending your knees further and rising up slowly one vertebrae at a time.

Where: Hips, hamstrings, upper and lower back.

When: You need a little blood flow after too much sitting.

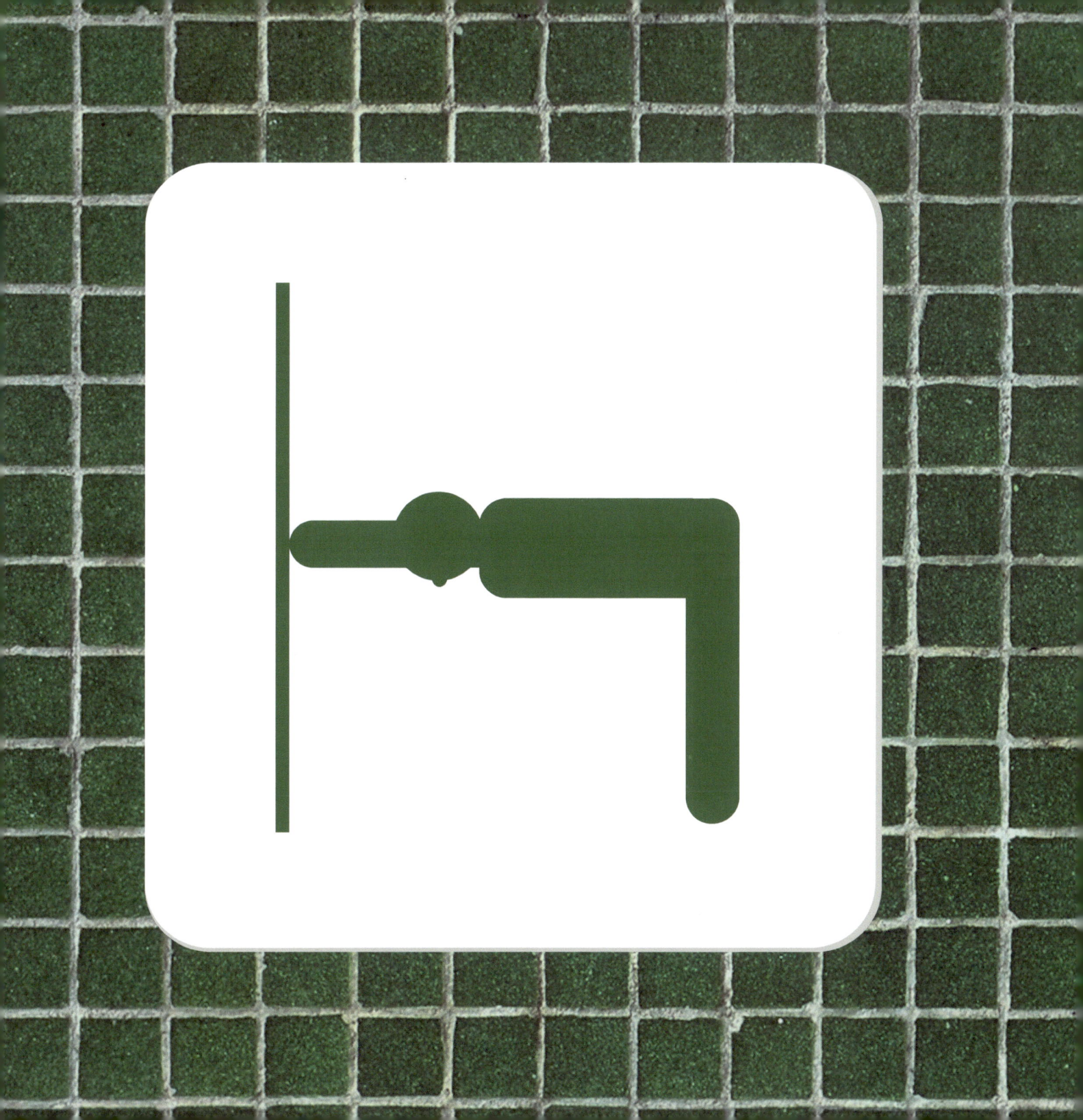

Forward Bend with Arm Wrap

- With your feet together or hip distance apart, bend your legs and bring your chest to your knees.

- Hug your legs, placing your arms on opposite elbows.

- Relax in this pose for 5 - 10 breaths. Avoid pulling yourself down and straining your back.

Where: Hips, hamstrings, upper and lower back.

When: You have been stationary and need to promote blood flow without a jog.

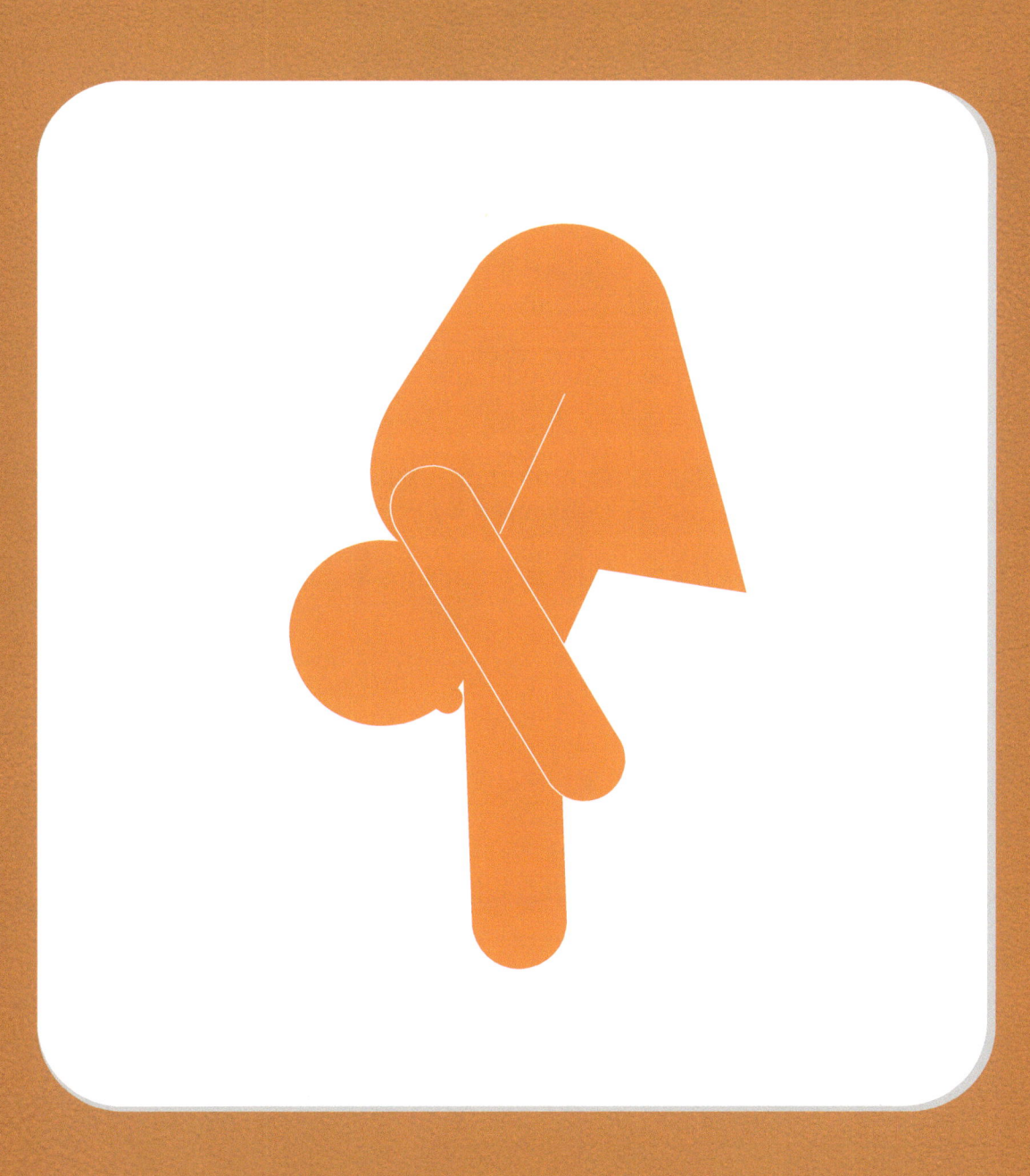

Chair

- Step your feet together until they are touching.

- On your next inhale, raise your arms up to the ceiling, keeping them shoulder distance apart.

- As you exhale, lower your butt back and down towards the ground, pressing your weight evenly through your feet.

- Lower down as far as is comfortable. Make sure that your toes are visible and not obscured by your knees.

- Hold this pose for 5 - 8 breaths, pushing deeper into the pose with each exhale.

Where: In every part of your legs, especially your butt and both sides of your thighs.

When: Your legs have started to fall asleep at your desk.

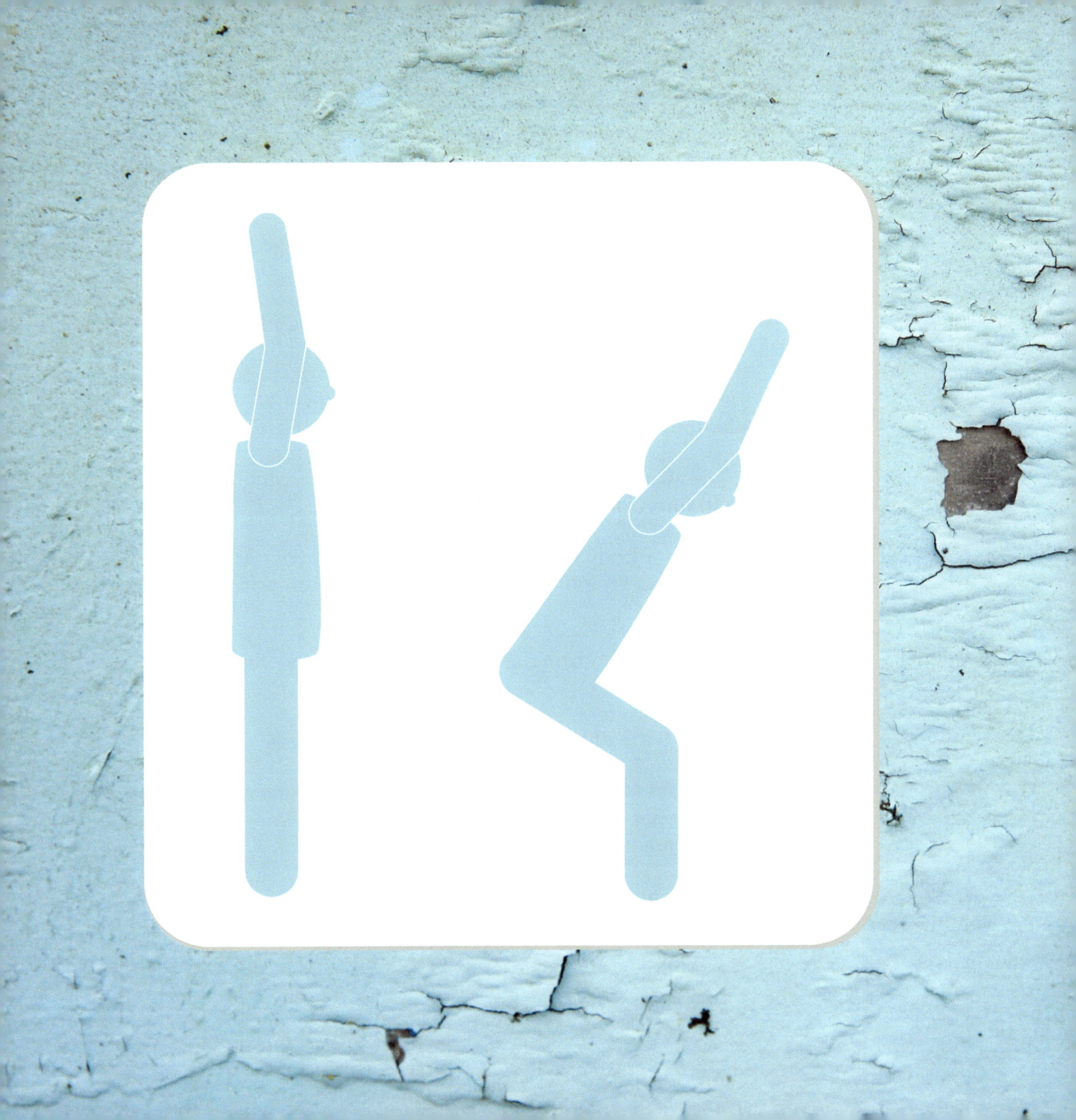

Runner's Lunge

- Start with your feet hip distance apart.

- Step your right leg straight back 3 to 4 feet, coming to rest on the toes of the foot with the heel up.

- Bend the opposite leg forward until the knee is over the ankle, forming a 90 degree angle.

- Maintain outward pressure with the front knee, keeping the kneecap in line with your 2 middle toes.

- With your upper body remaining upright, extend your arms up towards the ceiling or keep your palms together in front of your chest.

- For a deeper stretch push your hips forward, tucking your tailbone under.

- Hold for 5 - 10 breaths then step forward, switch legs and repeat.

Where: Front, upper and lower thighs
(hip flexor and quadriceps).

When: Your back and hips feel tight from sitting for too long.

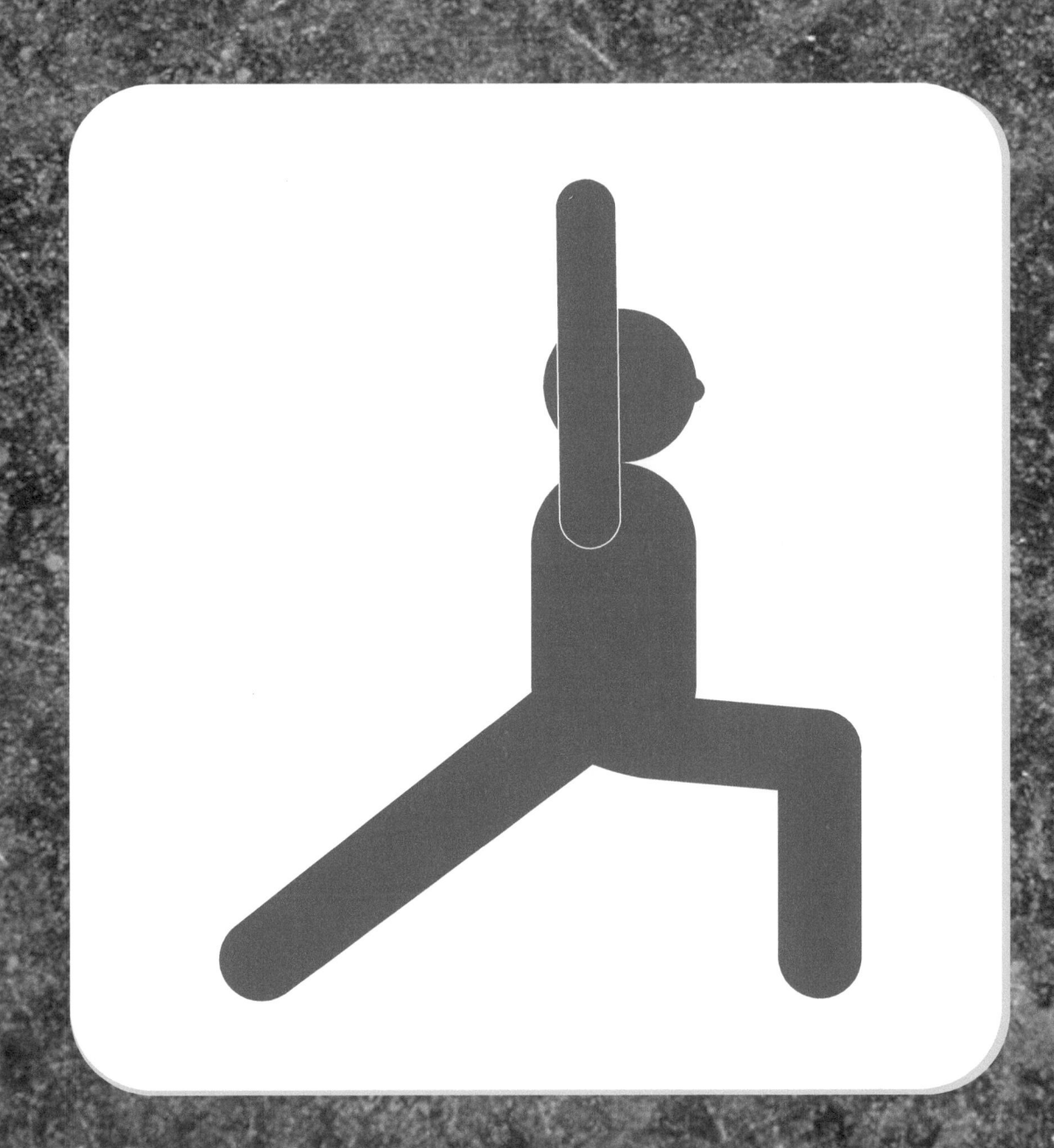

Modified Dancer

- Start with your feet together or slightly apart.

- Place your left hand on the wall in front of you for balance.

- Lift your right heel towards your butt and grab the top of your foot with your right hand.

- Standing up straight, keep both knees together and press your heel towards your butt.

- Hold for 5 - 10 breaths, then switch legs.

- Make certain to keep your hips in a neutral position to prevent back discomfort; avoid leaning forward or backward.

Where: Along your thighs, shins and feet.

When: Your hinges are stiff from sitting.

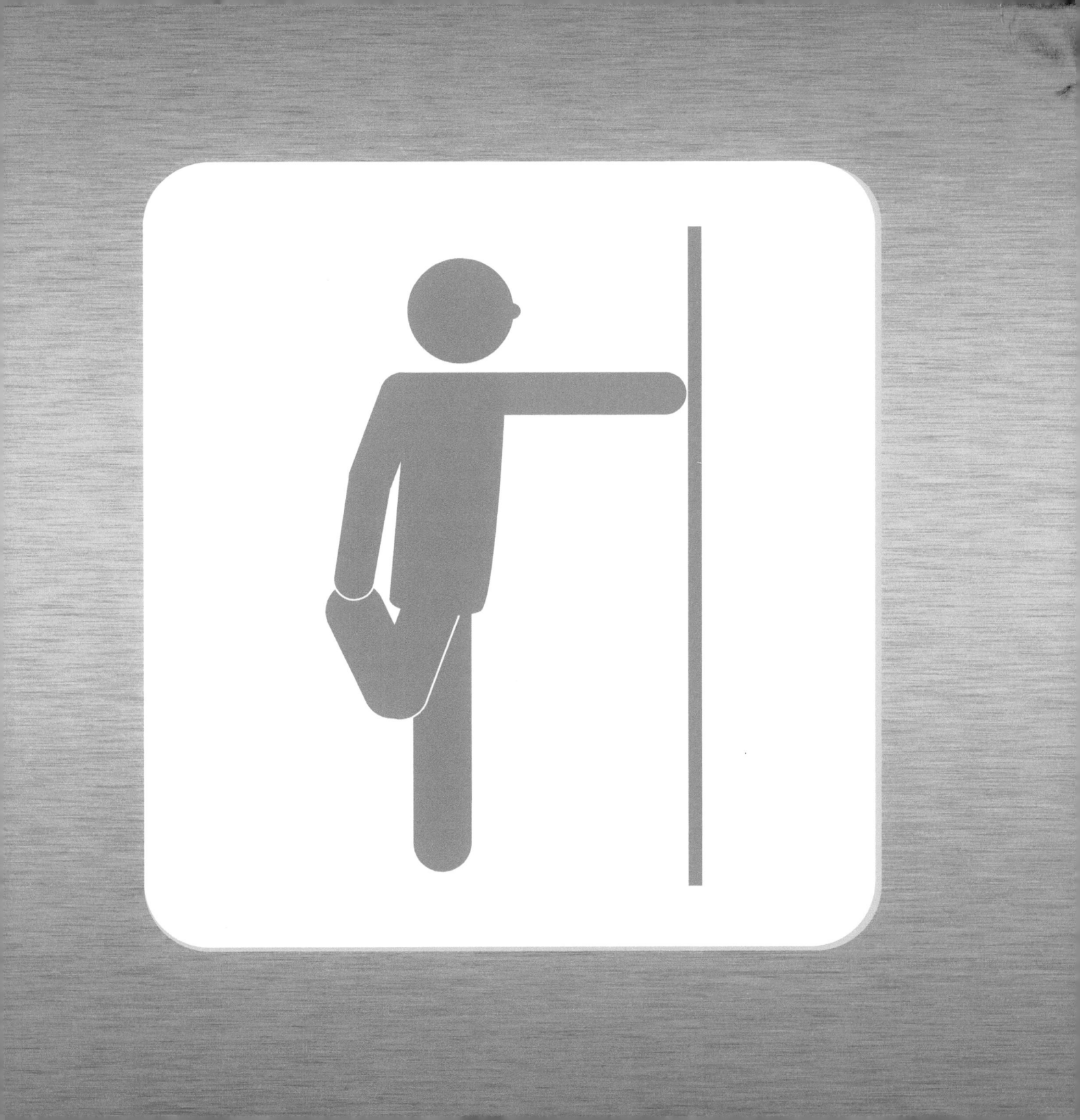

Biography

Grant Clark was born in New Jersey and attended Davidson College in North Carolina, where he met Rosie. Having studied Art, Grant completed his post-baccalaureate at Maryland Institute College of the Arts in Baltimore. In the meantime, he improved his health and chronic back pain by consulting a personal trainer, becoming interested in corrective exercises. Grant moved to San Francisco to obtain his Master's degree in painting at California College of the Arts. A year into his move, Rosie joined him. Once he completed his degree, they both moved to New Jersey where Grant continued to paint and became a personal trainer and yoga instructor.

Rosie Kosinski was born in England to Irish and Polish parents. Growing up in Jerusalem, Rosie attended an international school and was surrounded by the creativity of both parents. She immigrated to the U.S. and attended Davidson College, studying Art and French. Rosie moved to San Francisco and dabbled in illustration and graphic design. When Rosie and Grant moved to New Jersey, Rosie pursued her graphic design career as a freelance designer while continuing with painting and commissions.

For contact and information for Grant Clark please visit:
www.gcfitness.club or **www.grantclarkart.com**

For contact and information for Rosie Kosinski please visit:
www.shatteredpencil.com or **www.rosiekosinski.com**

www.ingramcontent.com/pod-product-compliance
Lightning Source LLC
Chambersburg PA
CBHW041829280526
45792CB00006B/2030